Healthier Lifestyle: Making the Transition

The Practical Guide to Healthy Living

By: Elaine Owens

9781630225810

TABLE OF CONTENTS

Elaine Owens

PUBLISHERS NOTES

Speedy Publishing LLC

40 E. Main St., #1156

Newark, DE 19711

www.speedypublishing.co

Cover Artwork: 24 Hr. Designs Ltd.

Editing: Speedy Publishing LLC

Book design: Speedy Publishing LLC

ISBN: 9781630225810

This is a reprint book.

DISCLAIMER

This publication is intended to provide helpful and informative material. It is not intended to diagnose, treat, cure, or prevent any health problem or condition, nor is intended to replace the advice of a physician. No action should be taken solely on the contents of this book. Always consult your physician or qualified health-care professional on any matters regarding your health and before adopting any suggestions in this book or drawing inferences from it.

The author and publisher specifically disclaim all responsibility for any liability, loss or risk, personal or otherwise, which is incurred as a consequence, directly or indirectly, from the use or application of any contents of this book.

Any and all product names referenced within this book are the trademarks of their respective owners. None of these owners have sponsored, authorized, endorsed, or approved this book.

Always read all information provided by the manufacturers' product labels before using their products. The author and publisher are not responsible for claims made by manufacturers.

DEDICATION

For Ruth - Keep trying. I have faith in you.

CHAPTER 1- ESTROGEN

Relationships can live longer, healthier, and happier if both parties conform their minds to think positively.

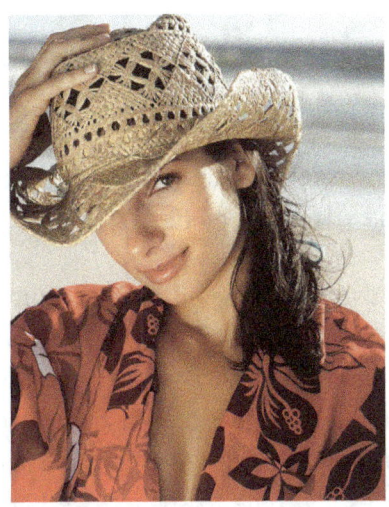

Did you know that women over the age 30 who have sex boost estrogen? All it takes is two times weekly, and your estrogen will boost. While we may discuss how you can live longer, healthier, and happier, we can talk about sex; since studies has proven that those actively enjoy sex live longer. In fact, nearly every song ever written revolves around sex. Why, well listen up.

Research has proven that women who engage in sexual acts more than twice per week has more estrogen count than those women who do not. Sex enforces exercise as well. When you have sex the pelvic muscles strengthen, which makes relaxation and muscle contraction easier. In addition, you work the entire body, which is adding activity to your life. In turn, you boost life, while feeling healthier and happier.

One of the largest problems in relationships today is that after spending so many years together, the sex drive diminishes. The reason is that most people think of sex at this point as a duty, rather than an enjoyment. I've had sex with you so many times, it always the same, says many. The fact is even if you've been together 30 years you can always make sex a new experience and enjoyment.

NOTE:

We are talking about partnership relationships, and not going out on the town and sleeping with multiple partners.

Relationships can live longer, healthier, and happier if both parties conform their minds to think positive. If you are used to having sex in the same position, or same area, why not switch up and do something different. A benefit to the people who spend years together, are that often the kids are grown and living their own life. The advantage gives you time to spend together in intimacy. Still, sex is more than spending time in the bedroom.

Sex is expressing feelings of love, candlelit dinners, long walks, holding hands, kissing, hugging, and so forth is all related to sex. When you show your partner that you love them, often you will feel happier, healthier, and will live longer.

Inactive sex is a leading reason why cheating, breakups, divorces, and so forth all occur. With this problem continuing, more and more people are unhappy. Thus, if you want to live longer, healthier, and happier, then including sex into your weekly schedule can bring you more than you hoped for.

Spicy Tips:

Elaine Owens

To promote sensuality, and intimacy you can set your moods. Light a few candles, share a glass of wine, and play a few romantic hits on the jukebox. Instead of having sex at the same time each day, change the pattern. For instance, if you often have sex at night time, switch to morning occasional.

Spending quality time together is the best solution for boosting relationships, and building happiness. When you spend quality time you set the mark that tells each other you care. In addition, instead of having sex in the bedroom often, take a U-turn and enjoy intimacy in the bathroom, kitchen, or the great outdoors. Think of each night as a new adventure instead of a "Let's get it over with attitude." In addition, you can talk walks together, which promotes exercise, as well as intimacy.

When you put forth positive thinking, you often live happier, as well your world will not crumble beneath you.

The benefits of intimacy can help you live longer, healthier, and happier, since it promotes good health, along with good relationships. Life is too short to stop living, thus women past the age 40 may think they are no longer attractive, but studies showed that older women are at the peaks of their life. Accepting menopause can also help you live longer, healthier, and happier.

CHAPTER 2- MENOPAUSE

Contrary to what other persons believe, menopause is not the end of a woman's life but merely a new chapter.

Menopause has affected millions of women down through the centuries, which many of the problems for menopause came from insufficient information and knowledge. The fact is menopause is a natural biological and physiological change that we cannot escape. Menopause has caused major stress problems, since misinformed in miscommunications has splattered abroad. Menopause is natural. There is nothing to worry about, you are not going to crawl in a hole and stop living. In fact, you could benefit from menopause. When a woman goes through menopause the biological clock stops ticking, as well, the menstrual cycle ceases. What a grand benefit. It gets better; you will not suffer PMS symptoms. NOTE: PMS include back and other bodily pains and aches and are not a mental issue.

Menopause in fact is the beginning of your life. Now don't get me wrong, you will experience hot flashes, heart palpitations, night sweats, mood swings, and drying in the vaginal area. The upside is that symptoms of menopause do not pose any risk to your health. You can reduce symptoms coming from menopause by practicing deep breathing. Deep breathing has proven to relieve women in menopause from symptoms up to 50 percent. You can also try to stay in a cool environment to minimize menopause symptoms.

One of the major problems that lead to stress is that down through the years people were taught that "the change" (Menopause) was the mark of the ending. You heard negative remarks such as, "Oh, she's going through the change." This remark alone put fear in many for years to come. The fact is you are now beginning to live.

Elaine Owens

You and I have to worry about your children, because likely they are grown and out of the house. You have the option of starting a new career, or advancing in your current career.

Menopause causes a woman's body to slow estrogen. What you can do to boost estrogen is incorporate soy into your diet, and has sex more than twice a week.

Some women endure depression, and mood swings that cause them to lash out. While no proof is available that links these behaviors to menopause, some studies believe that night sweats and hot flashes has something to do with it. The fact is chemical imbalance, as well as other mental reasons may underlie the problem. You may need mental health assistance to cope. One thing you can do when you feel down and out, is to pamper yourself, reward yourself, and try to avoid belittling yourself.

To live longer, healthier, and happier you want to include exercise into your daily plans. Studies and proven that exercise, such as walking, can increase chemicals and endorphins which will make you feel better both inside and out. Exercise will improve mood swings, as well as strengthen in your muscles to prevent osteoporosis. In addition, stretch exercises will promote flexibility, mobility, and spare your joints from harm.

Women going through menopause are candidates for osteoporosis, simply because estrogen decreases. Again sex promotes estrogen; accordingly you want to learn to train the mind to enjoy your partner.

To live longer and healthier, as well as happier you also want to learn to relax the body and mind. Taking time out for you is essential in promoting good health.

Healthier Lifestyle: Making the Transition
Now that you've learnt that menopause is not a bad thing, you can move ahead by accepting changes. Those who accept change, has proven to live longer, healthier, and happier. Change is good. Change is your friend. Change is what helps us to live and grow.

CHAPTER 3- CHANGES

If you want to live longer, healthier, and happier you have to turn those bad habits into good habits and continue living in harmony with the change.

Change is what makes us grow through transformations, which modify the way we live. Change is a revolutionized expression or action that helps us to adjust and amend problems. Many people fear change, yet the fact is change is your best friend. The only way change can hurt you, is you allowing the emotions to take control and continuing fearing change.

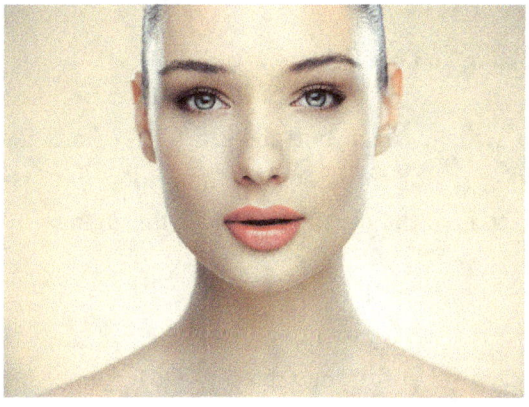

People, who cannot accept change, often resort to bad habits, such as alcoholism, drugs, smoking, prostitution, crime, promiscuous behaviors, and so forth. All of these bad habits lead to poor health, death, and misery.

The problem reaches far and wide, since those who cannot accept change reflect their behaviors on others. The saying, "Misery loves company," is more factual and you realize.

Accordingly if you want to live longer, healthier, and happier you have to turn those bad habits into good habits and continue living in harmony with the change. The fact is you're going to go through problems in life. Problems are unavoidable. You cannot escape problems. You have to learn to live with problems, grow with problems, and except change.

One of the leading problems why people cannot accept change is that down through the century's lies, miscommunication, and misunderstandings has made people believe that change is an enemy. To help you better understand change, we can give you up you helpful tips, so that you can transform your mind until positive direction. When you live a positive life, i.e. when you think positive you reflect sheer energy that brings in rewards.

Tips for Relating To Change:

Change is a switch, which buttons are hit. We call them triggers. Change challenges or threatens the emotions, yet the underlying cause is due to how the person perceives the change.

Positive:

The change is a substitute or replacement for what I once knew, I will live and grow with it.

Negative:

When the emotions are scared, or challenged the person will often act out in anger, or express pessimistic thoughts, or may feel anxious, nervous, and panicky. Often when change occurs a person will act out negative, since that person may lack resources that can help him or her find a solution to the problem.

For instance, people often experience debt problems, which too many times they fail to see a way out. A helpful tip can send you in the right direction. Visit your library and the Internet to learn more about debt solutions.

Tip:

Did you know that few people fear change so severely, that they will keep the same hairstyle for years?

One of the best solutions for growing to accept change is to practice changing your lifestyle. You can start with exercise and diet. Tell you now that each day you plan to take a 30 minute walk. At the end of the week record your results and consequences.

Instead of eating greasy chicken, change your dish to baked chicken. Baked skinless chicken is much healthier.

If you watch television more than 3 hours daily, plan to cut back on time consumed in entertainment, instead visit a friend and enjoy social activities.

If you keep your hair styled one way, try something new. Each step you take to accept change will lead you to a brighter and healthier future.

Tip:

Did you know that what you put in your mind comes out in your habits and behaviors. If you watch programs that include violence, nudity, strong language, and so on, it will show later in your future. These are proven unhealthy practices that are destined to kill the entire race of people. Relaxation and sleep is also essential for living longer and healthier.

CHAPTER 4- RELAXATION AND SLEEP

Exercise will eliminate excessive amounts of stress, even if you work a 60 hour shift.

When you do not get enough rest or relaxation it affects the body and mind. Often you will feel frustrated, tired, hopeless, moody, and so forth. One of the major problems today is insomnia, sleeping disorders, and so forth. Millions of people every night struggle to get proper rest. One of the problem is many people find it difficult to relax the body and mind. Often people will go to bed worrying about how they are going to pay their next bill, or else worrying about something that has happened yet. Many people also go to bed angry.

Now we see a problem that is causing major health issues and even death. To help you learn to live longer, healthier, and happier, we are going to discuss exercise, stress reducers, acceptance, diet, supplements, and so forth.

Exercises are at the top of the list. Millions of people in the world do not daily perform activities and move the muscles and stretches the joints. For this reason, people are undergoing high-volumes of stress level, which is becoming the leading cause of death.

Nowadays, people are so obsessed with surviving that often they will overwork themselves. Millions of people spend more time and work in what they do at home. This is the leading reason stress is escalating, families are dying, and increasing problems is unfolding.

It is essential that you exercise, find quality time to spend with family, and self, as well as move to a healthier living. Exercise is a stress reducer. Exercise will eliminate excessive amounts of stress, even if you work a 60 hour shift.

When you exercise you learn to accept through appreciation that life has more to offer than battling sleep and relaxation. When you include diet and supplements to your daily exercise schedule, you increase relaxation, sleep, and a healthier way of living.

Now we can discuss a few mental tactics that will help you seize worrying, which will also promote sleep and relaxation.

Tips:

When you say every day, "Sufficient each day, for no man knows what tomorrow will bring," you are training the mind to cease worry, and to focus on the here and now.

When you say, "One day at a time," you are saying, sufficient for each day. Learning to take it one day at a time can help you live longer, healthier, and happier.

Remember to change the things you can change, and let God change the things you cannot change. Furthermore, worrying about something that has occurred yet is only setting yourself up for a fall.

Tip:

If you focus on one task at a time you can reduce stress. Thinking of more than one task can lead to frustration. Handle the first task and then move onto the next.

Due to advances in technology, the Internet and television is consuming more time of many and any other thing in the world. If you surf the Internet and late hours, or watch television more than three hours a day, you are building stress. The body needs more activity than it needs to sit around.

Healthier Lifestyle: Making the Transition

While preparing for bed, always prepare to rest at the same time each night. This will help you sleep and relax. You may want to change your bedroom around to promote a restful environment. Do not sit around looking at the clock when you prepare for bed. If you find it hard to sleep after lying down for an hour or so, get up and do something, such as exercise. Relaxation and sleep is essential for living longer, healthier, and happier. You can rest better when you learn the steps to reduce stress.

CHAPTER 5- REDUCING STRESS

It is important to learn how to reduce stress.

Stress is the leading cause of various illnesses, and today stress if becoming one of the largest killers in the world. The first thing you need to be aware of before you can work to live longer, healthier, and happier, is the signs of stress. Knowing the signs can help you fight back, and win the nasty battle. Stress includes early warnings (Prevention time), mental symptoms, emotional symptoms, physiologic or physical symptoms, and behavioral symptoms.

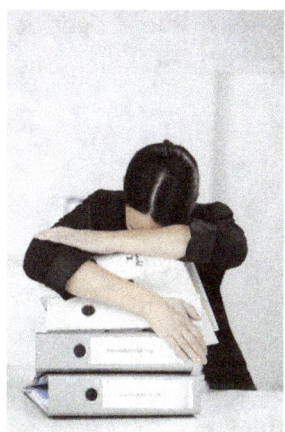

The Signs:

Prevention Time:

When you start to feel irritable often, and your patience is thin you are walking on the fine lines of stress. Often the irritability moves to edgy feelings, uptight or tension, and aggressive behaviors. The person may snap each time someone speaks to them, thus acting out angrily. The aggressiveness turns to oversensitivity, which leads to easiness in taking offense against what others say and do, as well the person will blame others for his or her problems, and often express moodiness.

The mind thinks pessimistically, which turns to a feeling of tiredness and restlessness. At this point stress increases, which leads to inability to sleep, overeating, or under eating. The feelings increase to changes in diet, which often leads to unhealthy eating. The person may start to depend on alcohol, drugs, or cigarettes to cope. The feeling brings in nausea, upset stomach, constipation, and/or diarrhea. The symptoms increase to nervousness, twitching, and form into habits such as biting the nails, pulling hair, itching, or jiggling the knees.

If you notice one or more of these signs, it is time to take action now. You can start with exercise, diet, and socialization to avoid further complications.

Mental Signs:

If the signs go unnoticed, or left without attention, mental signs develop, which include inability to concentrate. In turn the person forgets often. The person may feel confused often, and find it hard to make easy decisions. The perspective follows pursuit, i.e. the person is unable to think clearly, which leads to obsession. The person will feel a nagging sensation, thus stressing over time. The signs lead to mental burnouts or exhaustion.

If you are at this level, again exercise, diet, and supplements can help you reduce stress. You may also want to seek professional help.

Emotional Signs;

Once the signs appear, and the mental indicators develop the emotional response begins to decline. Rather, the emotions will act out by showing increasing levels of panic attacks and anxiety. The emotions will strike by diminishing the self-esteem, and will move to depression and pessimistic thinking. You feel hopeless.

The emotions then move to feelings of anger, while harboring resentment. This makes the person moody, which forces tears to flow for no apparent reason. The person will find it hard to laugh, and will undergo frequent nightmares.

At this point you need immediate help. While I am not against mental health services, I can say these people lack wisdom and experience in many lands, thus walk with precaution when seeking mental help. Get out of the house more, exercise, and diet, which will help you, fight the emotional stimulus.

Physical Signs:

Once the emotional responses develop showing signs of stress, the body will experience agony. This is where health problems start to show. The muscular fatigue and tension makes it difficult to think, which adds additional stress. The body will start to feel aches in the back, shoulders, and neck. (Chiropractic Services has proven to reduce stress stemming from physical signs of stress) Once the body aches, the eyes start to feel tired. The muscles begin to twitch, especially near the corner of the eyes. Your mouth feels dry, and often your jaw will feel locked. The palms begin to sweat, and the fingers feel cool. You start to experience heartburn and indigestion, as well as feeling the need to urinate more often. The signs continue to bladder infections, and move on to you feel breathless. Once you feel breathlessness, your breathing starts too erratic or hyperventilates. The heart begins to palpitate, and finally you feel headaches and frequent colds taking over your soul. The problems increase, since you start to gain or lose weight, and finally the libido feels lost and its impotency has blundered.

We now have serious risks of disease. Still, there is more to come.

Behavioral Signs:

Now that your mind and body has lost control, you begin to lash out in anger while showing aggression. (Criminal-based potential) You begin talking without cease, since the thoughts are racing like cars around the India 500. With talking excessively, you begin to cut others off who are speaking. You show nervous habits, which include tapping the fingers, pulling the hair, biting the nails, or jiggling the knees. The only outing you see at this time is to consume yourself in work; you become a workaholic, and often feel absenteeism from the rest of the world. This brings us to isolation. You start to withdraw socially, and move toward neglecting personal hygiene. You now have a serious problem, since you develop obsessive-compulsive behaviors, which include excessive hand washing, monitoring the doors and windows often and so forth.

If your problems have escalated to this level, you need mental health now. It's time to take the steps to reduce stress.

CHAPTER 6- STEPS TO REDUCE STRESS

It is up to you to find the best diet that works for you, which can help you live a healthier lifestyle..

One of the ways to reduce stress is to understand the principals of eating a balanced diet. Reducing stress is essential in living healthier, longer, and happier. If you fail to reduce stress heart disease may walk in your door and kick your butt. In addition, if you fail to reduce stress you can put the body at risk of cancer, diabetes, high-blood, high-cholesterol, and so forth. Fighting now is the only way you can survive and live a longer, healthier, and happier life. The steps to reducing stress to live longer, healthier, and happier include:

Diet:

It is essential to eat three balanced meals daily, or spread the meals out to five small portions daily. While eating you should avoid digesting the food quickly, rather take your time and allow the food to process in the digestive system. You want to include five helpings of fruits and vegetables in your daily plan. Drinking one a glass of water one half before and after meals can help you maintain weight.

Preparing to live longer, healthier and happier, includes a balanced diet. Still, you need stretch exercise and exercise routines to live longer.

Posture:

Keeping the posture straight can help you avoid bone related disease. When the posture is straight you will promote free breathing, which relieves stress. A straight posture will also promote energy and vitality, which is essential for living longer. Straight postures will also promote relaxation, since your head is supported. In addition, a straight posture will increase confidence, as well as make you look youthful, in shape, and slimmer.

Activities:

Regular exercise will make you relax and sleep with fewer problems. Exercise will enhance your energy, while raising yourself-esteem and confidence. You will look and feel great. A general schedule should include 20 to 30 minutes daily of activities.

Exercise will also work at a couple of minutes at a time. If you have problems getting started, start exercise slowly and gradually work into a full routine.

Sleep:

Each night go to bed at the same hour. Sleep will reduce stress. You will need to change your bedroom if you find it difficult to sleep at night. A change can make you feel more at ease. You should also keep the room dark and quiet during sleep hours. Avoid naps, unless you suffer illnesses. Make sure that your mattress and pillow fits your posture and makes you feel at ease. Do not use caffeine, smoke, or drink before going to bed. You can workout one hour before bedtime to achieve tiredness. If you often awake during night hours, get out of bed when you find it difficult to sleep and read a book.

Training the Mind:

Train your mind to relax and think positive. Train your mind to think only during wake hours. Try to focus on one task at a time, which will promote memory and relaxation. Do not worry, rather do something about it.

Breathing and Relaxing:

Become aware of your breathing and move to breathe properly. This will help you relax.

Meditate Daily:

Mediation is enlightenment of the spiritual mind. When you meditate properly you practice straight posture, breathing, focus, and attitude.

Stretch Exercise:

Stretching can help you to flex the joints, which promotes strong muscles. Stretching will open the airways, and help you to feel relaxed. To help you get started we can post a few positions.

Position 1: Sun Salutation Stretch:

Stand straight up with your feet coming together. Bring the palms to the front of your chest and breathe.

Breathing in; now, stretch the arms over the head and bend slightly backwards, while the palms face forward. Breathe outward, and bend the body forward, while placing the palms of your hands flat on the floor at the sides of your feet. Lower your face to the knees as closely as possible, and stretch up into position.

Next, we can look at a few potential dietary facts.

Dietary Facts in How to Live Longer and Healthier

Growing to a happier future

Millions of people eat foods daily that they believe helps them to live longer and healthier. Yet few facts are hidden, which will prove them wrong. In this article I am going to tell you foods to avoid, which will help you live healthier. Keep in mind, new information come available daily, and the facts are constantly changing. Therefore, this is not a concrete guide that you should listen to. Talk to your doctor to learn more about foods, but most will tell you to stick with fruits, vegetables and salads for a healthier living.

Facts:

Lunch meats and packaged sausage has proven to present health risks. The products contain what experts know as nitrates. Nitrates are a chemical radical or compound that includes salt and ester. As well, the products include nitric acids, which contain radical NO3. The preservatives help supermarkets to store the products longer than a few days. (Nitrates is utilized in fertilizers also) The products also have additives.

Some of the products you want to be aware of are bratwurst, Italian sausage, liver sausage, turkey and pork sausage, Braunschweiger, duck sausage, and so forth.

According to experts you should avoid buying hormone, antibiotic-free, and range fed poultry and meats. What you want to avoid is veal, quail, pheasant, squab, pork, duck, lamb, chicken, beef, and so forth. (NOTE: The information is based on resources that fall under the Schwarzben principles)

Cheese:

The better cheeses available include, cream, cottage cheese, goat, feta, Neufchatel, Queso fresco, Mozzarella, Gjetost, Muenster, and Ricotta.

Elaine Owens
Facts:

Smoked fish often contains nitrates.

Protein based foods:

Shellfish and fish:

Saturated vs. unsaturated fats:

According to studies avoiding saturated fats can help you live longer, healthier, and happier. New studies have proven otherwise. According to resources when the studies were conducted to test the results of saturated fats, thus the majority were eating unhealthy, smoking, drinking excessively, using drugs, and so forth. New studies where the people were living healthier showed that saturated fats can improve cholesterol. As well, saturated fats can decrease the blood pressure, as well as reduce heart disease.

Facts;

Excess Intakes of carbohydrates will increase the level of insulin. The balanced diet should include 50 to 80 grams of carbohydrates daily. You should also eat carbohydrates that include fats and proteins.

Eating whole grain foods, as fruits and vegetables with starch and legumes is healthier than carbohydrates made by man.

Facts:

Crackers have additives, which may include hydrogenate fats.

Recommended serving:

Whole Wheat Matzo crackers: one half

Rice Crackers; no more than 4 crackers

Rusk toast: 1 ½ ounce

Rice cakes: 2 cakes

One thing you want to keep in mind while considering diet is that diets are like fads. Everyone seems to think they have the answer to living healthy through diet, yet only your body knows what it needs. I recommend you take note and pay attention to your body's demand. If your body agrees with the food it may be the answer to your prayers. On the other hand, if your body disagrees you may want to find a new food to test.

One of the foods on the marketplace low in fat is Chinese food. Most people believe that fat makes you fat, but the fact is our body needs a measure of fat to survive. We need balance. Fats build hormones, cells, and components of the brain. Since, fats do not stimulate release of insulin, thus fats is not what makes you fat. Overall, it is up to you to find the best diet that pleases your body, which can help you live healthier. Learning more about the secrets of diet can help you live longer, healthier, and happier.

CHAPTER 7- SECRETS OF DIET

Another problem is dieters fail to stick with a plan. This is why many gain weight.

The world is filled with people who tell you to avoid eating this, or eat this to live longer. Most diet plans are like cars, i.e. they are out dated before you know it. No, wait a minute. Diet plans is like superstition, over the years the lies add up and after a while millions believes that if they eat particular foods they will curl up and die. The fact is only you know what is best for your body. What people need to do is listen to their body's and let the ruler take control.

For the most part you can eat pretty much anything you like as long as you exercise. The key is adhering to balanced diets. Exercise is the ruler, which if you exercise, no matter what you do you can increase life. Still, you want to avoid harmful things that will lead to poor health. One of the worst things you can do is stop and start exercise. When you start, keep going.

To help you understand more about diet however, we can consider a few expert tips. According to experts if you eat five helpings of fruits and vegetables daily, you will expend your life. NOTE: Juicers blended from juicers can reduce the intake of fruits and vegetables, which will save you money; as well the juices will give you twice the amount of nutrients you will get from a single fruit or vegetable.

Fruits and vegetables are high, thus who can truly afford to eat five helpings daily, yet the fact is fruits and vegetables is the healthier produce, since it comes from natural resources.

Funny:

According to some experts eating too much fruits and vegetables can make you gain weight. The experts tell you to eat only half an apple a day, while superstitious beliefs lead people to believe that an apple a day will keep the doctor away.

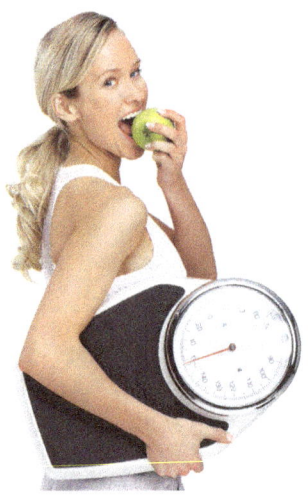

One of the leading causes of weight gain is the not food you eat, rather it is the obsession behind the person. People obsess over gaining weight, rather than eat according to the body's signals. Thus the only truth that come from diet experts this far is those that tell you to listen to your body. If your body tells you it is hungry, eat. If your body says it's full, stop eating. If your body tells you it needs something, give your body what it needs.

Obsessive eaters often gain weight, since they stress over weight gain rather than taking action to do something about. Often they will ignore their body signals and go on a binge eating plan. When the body is full, the obsessive eater will continue eating, thus disregarding the signals of the body, which adds to deeper problems.

Another problem is dieters fail to stick with a plan. They will often jump track and binge eat, or will not eat at all. They will also change the balance of their diet. This is why many gain weight.

Another problem that leads to poor health is that many obsessive eaters will degrade their being. When you spend time degrading self, such as "I am fat," you are wasting valuable time that could help you achieve a healthier living. The people, who achieve good health, thus are often instinctive eaters.

Now you have it. It is up to you to start reading the signals of your body to learn what it needs. It is up to you to attend to your bodily needs. Therefore, stop worrying over weight and start learning how you can live healthier, longer, and happier. Instinctive eaters often live longer than those who obsess over food.

CHAPTER 8- INSTINCTIVE EATERS

Instincts are a natural biological drive, which sets a pattern of behaviors.

Dieting information spreads throughout the lands and everyone has their own idea as to what plan is best to lose weight, live longer, and feel happier. The fact is all diets can work for you, yet you must understand what your body needs, and the way to do this is listen to your body talk. The world has two types of eaters, i.e. the obsessive eaters and the instinctive eaters. The instinctive eaters often fare better than obsessive eaters. Instinctive eaters will eat as they like, yet they know when it is time to stop. Learning the difference between obsessive eaters and instinctive eaters can help you see how one can live longer than the other one.

Instinctive eaters listen to their body talk. The healthy people will know when the body is hungry, know when the body is content, and know what the body wants. Only your body can tell you what it truly needs. Once you learn to adapt your thinking, you can move to healthier living.

Instincts are a natural biological drive, which sets a pattern of behaviors. The goal of instincts is to survive and reproduce. Instincts are a powerful impulse reaction, which acts on natural feelings, rather than he said, she said. It is a natural gift and skill, which unfortunately is diminishing throughout the years.

Instinctive eaters will not abuse, struggle, deprive, or adhere to a diet. The fact is diets can become dangerous, insulting, and most are unnatural.

Secrets Revealed:

At the moment, dietary industries are spending billions of dollars each year to prevent you from learning that diets often do not work.

The first step to restoring your natural instincts to prevent you from falling ill to diets is to learn to accept your body. Once you learn to accept your body, naturally you will start to see where your next step leads you. Obsessive eaters often fail in losing weight, since they are too busy worrying about how to lose weight, and often they will beat their self-esteem down into the mud.

Fact:

Most women believe that if they cannot wear a size six in clothing, they are fat.

The truth:

This is far from the truth.

Fact:

Media, television, magazines, have all programmed people to believe there is something wrong with them if they do not fit the model profile.

Truth:

This is a lie, since many models are superficial.

The best rule of thumb when working to live healthier, longer, and happier is to realize who you are and accept it. If you learn to use your natural instincts to guide your way, you will eat what you want, when you want, and how much you want. Still, you must listen to the signals of your body.

Natural instincts will put the brakes on those misconstrued influenced beliefs, which comes from dietary experts, and media, and lead you to feeling positive about food. In other words, food will become a friend, rather than a fear. You will no longer overeat or under eat.

Listening to your instincts will help you to avoid anorexia and bulimia. As you grow to healthier living you will soon handle your emotions well, which will reduce stress. When you learn to accept who you are, you will not avoid clothes you like to wear; rather you will jump in them and go. Instinctive eaters often respect their body and mind, which moves you to living healthier, happier, and longer. When you conform to natural ways of good health, and listen to your body you will lose weight under a natural program, and it will require little effort on your part. You will also avoid depriving the body of what it needs. New breakthroughs are showing a better way to live longer and happier.

CHAPTER 9- THE BREAKTHROUGHS

If you learn to use natural instincts you can lose weight without dieting.

Those who believe they have a problem losing weight, is only convincing themselves that they have a problem. If you want to lose weight you need to transform your way of thinking. One of the largest problems with people trying to lose weight is they never believe any weight is ideal. They will sometimes say, "I am overweight and there is nothing I can do about it." Wrong, you can do something about it and it takes you to transform the mind and work to achieve. One of the biggest breakthroughs in dieting comes from the "Body-Signal Program." This program transforms your mind to think naturally, which has proven to help you live longer, healthier, and happier, as you lose weight.

The fact is diet plans are gimmicks that has set you up for major falls. Most diet ads send out messages that put you in fear. For instance, the ad may show a sexy female with a heavenly body, yet what they don't tell you is this person is a show and tell. The female you see also experiences episodes of fear, thus terrified she will gain weight. Why, because we are set up as competitors to glory and fame, which lead us to believe that if we do not look like Pam Anderson or Cindy Crawford, we are a failure. The fact is we are not the failures; we have failed because millions of lies have filled our minds.

The truth is God gave us naturally instincts, which if we listen to the communication it sends, we can successfully do anything we want. Although, society and the media have diminished instincts, we can transform back to natural thinking. The body also sends out signals, which if you take the time to listen to and understand you can grow to a healthier lifestyle.

The breakthroughs are showing that dietary industries are spending billions each year to prevent you from learning the facts about diets. Diets do not work, they may say because you did not stick with the plan. The fact is the diet probably never worked anyway.

New breakthroughs are showing that if you learn to use natural instincts you can lose weight without dieting, using diet pills, or falling into snares that gimmicks often deliver. This is the only true source of living healthier programs that I have seen on the market. Through natural instincts you will listen to your body when it tells you what you need.

Rather than allow the fears that built up over the years from scores of diet plans, let your fears go and learn what your body needs. Doctors, mental health experts, diet experts, and so forth are mere helpers, yet these people cannot tell you more than you already know about your body and mind. Of course, if you have diabetes, thus a doctor comes in handy.

When you learn to let go and let God's natural sources step in, you will feel free to do whatever you desire within reason. Learning to stop listening to those gimmicks will put you in control, since you will learn to accept who you are. This is one of the major problems, is that many do not accept.

Still, once you learn to adhere to natural thinking and listen to signals of the body, you will need exercise. Exercise is an added benefit, and no matter what you eat you will lose weight, feel good, and live longer. If you cannot see what follows, and then consider that feeling good brings forth happiness. The power of acceptance can bring you many rewards.

CHAPTER 10- THE POWER OF ACCEPTANCE

When you learn to accept you and allow body signs and instincts guide your path, you will live longer, healthier, and happier life.

Acceptance is a power that allows you to see who you are. When you learn to accept, you learn to grow. When you start to grow you learn what it takes to live longer, healthier, and happier. The power of acceptance gives you recognition that promotes favorable receptions. The opposite of acceptance is rejection, which leads to denial.

Now you may wonder what this has to do with living longer, healthier, and happier, but acceptance has everything in the world with a better future. Most people are obsesses with good health and weight control, and most are obsessing simple because they read all the lies that tell them how to lose weight. The fact is no diet in the world is going to help you lose weight; this is why diets come and go. Only natural eaters enjoy the benefits of living healthier, longer, and happier.

Weight problems are people who hinder their life by obsessing, rather than enjoying what life has to offer. SO what if you weigh 200 pounds, if you learn to accept your body, and allow your natural instincts to move obstacles that hinder you from listening to your body signals, thus you will lose 20 pounds in a few weeks or months.

The problem is with weight; rather the problem is how people think. For the most part women tend to fall into a fad, i.e. they strive to look like a supermodel. They often see these pretty women on television, and work hard to look like them. If these women stopped, and started accepting self they may find a beautiful woman stepping out into a brighter future.

The way many men has acted, along with media, magazines, and many misleading writes, thus people conform to obsession believing they have to be something they are not. Acceptance of who you are is the only way you are going to see through the many blind folds put up in front of you.

Now, if you want to learn what it takes to live longer, healthier, and happier. Then stop obsessing, start accepting that you are, and get up and do something about it. Exercise is the ONLY, ONLY, source that will provide your life-sustaining forces that will guide you to healthier living.

When you learn to accept you and allow body signs and instincts guide your path, as well as start exercising...BAM, you will live longer, healthier, and happier.

Fact:

Those overweight often fail to see that thin people also obsess over weight.

Yes, it is true. So happens, I was one of those people and what happen to me was, I gained weight and later realized that I should had appreciated what I had then. My body was great, and instead of obsessing I could had accepted and today I would not be looking back, rather I would feel healthier about me. Still, there is time, and starting today is the answer, since it is never too late to start working toward better health.

People often try to avoid fat foods, since they have been told so many stories, including fat foods make you gain weight. The fact is,

Elaine Owens

fats are essential to the body, and what make you gain weight are the highs and lows of insulin.

The truth of foods however is that FDA is allowing additives and harmful chemicals into our foods that before long, no food will be healthy to eat. The bible called it, "Man is bringing injury to self." Still, you can live longer by learning to listen to your natural instincts. Learning what to avoid can help you live happier.

CHAPTER 11- WHAT TO AVOID

Listen to your body and allow it to guide you to freedom- don't become one of the many that sit in a fantasy trying to be someone they are not

At what time working to live happier, healthier, and longer you want to avoid thinking negative or setting yourself up for falls. You will also need to avoid those misleading slicks that tell you the proper diet plan was discovered and we guarantee you will lose weight and feel healthier.

Avoiders:

You should never allow anyone other than yourself to tell you what you look like, i.e. do not allow them to set your appearance. Only you know what looks best for you.

You want to avoid idealism, i.e. do not let anyone misguide you. If you are overweight, accept it and allow your natural instincts to guide you.

Learn to listen to your body. At what time your body feels hungry eat a balanced meal, and when your body has had enough, stop eating.

Learn to love yourself, and stop looking for points about you to pick on. In other words, do not sit around telling yourself that you need to change this or that because it is unattractive. Learn to accept you are different and unique.

You want to avoid diet plans or advertisements that mislead you. The truth is no diet plan will help you until you learn to accept who you are. Still, if you listen, the body's natural instincts it will guide you to good health.

You want to avoid obsessing over weight. Diet advertisements have sent people on binges, and have caused them to fail many times, simply because the dieters did not listen to what their body needs.

Learn to focus. At what time you stay focused on living healthier, happier, and longer, you will strive to succeed. When you stay focus you will instill motivation that will drive you home.

You want to avoid sabotage thinking, such as "I can't do it, I'm too fat." Sabotage thinking only leads to poor health. You cannot live longer, healthier, or happier if you do not think positive.

To live longer, healthier, and happier you want to learn how to master your emotions by using your mind to think. Emotions are master destroyers of health, and the reason often comes from misleading information over the years, "Emotions are bad." Emotions are friends if you allow them to be your friend. Take charge of your life now!

At what time you work to live healthier, longer, and happier you learn to disconnect your commitments from your emotions. In other words, do not associate exercise as a commitment, rather view exercise as your friend.

You want to avoid overeating and to do this you can listen to the hungry pangs your body sends. You also want to avoid the slicks that claim they have discovered the best diet plan that works. You want to recognize your commitments that will help you remain faithful to you.

Acceptance is the ultimate key to moving toward healthier, happier, and longer living. When you learn to accept who you are, you start to love yourself.

Overall, there is no diet plan that will send you to perfection. If you want to lose weight, learn to be yourself and allow room for living and growing. Millions of people are sitting in a fantasy trying to be someone they are not. This is negative thinking that sends them on fat-mobile, and down misery lane. The lane is often crowded, thus it will lead you to poor health and an early death. Take charge now and listen to your body and allow it to guide you to freedom.

CHAPTER 12- OBSESSIVE EATERS

Knowing the difference between your optimal weight and ideal weight can help you lose weight.

Obsessive eaters act out on compulsions, which sometimes lead them to fanatical thinking. They become fixed or infatuated with an idea, which leads them to neurotic behaviors. The behaviors often include binge eating, starvation, excessive drinking, drugs, smoking, and so forth. Sometimes the compulsions send them straight to jail.

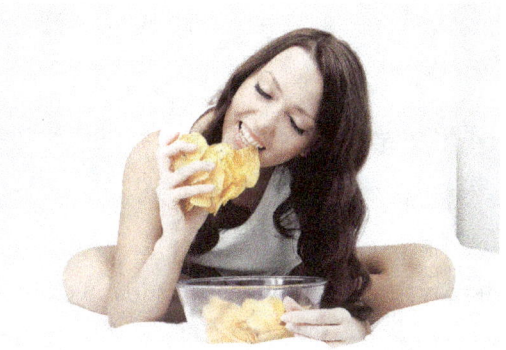

If you are searching for a way to live longer, healthier, and happier stop worrying about looking like someone else, rather learn to look like you. When you accept who you are, you are moving to healthier living.

One of the best ways to control weight is listening to your body, and allowing it to guide you to good health. When the body says it's hungry, then feed the body. When to body says it's had enough, stop eating. Simple strategies will help you lose weight.

To control obsessive eating you can train mind and body to eat properly. You can start by taking your time and enjoy your full, rather than guzzle it down. This is a huge problem that leads to obesity.

Instead of worrying about what you eat, learn to listen to natural instincts that will guide you in the right direction. If you think, or believe that diet is the answer, then think again. The fact is down to the centuries with each diet plan that has ever been advertised, all were quickly pushed to back when you diet plan came into focus. The truth is there is no diet pill, nor diet that will help you lose weight and keep the weight off.

To lose weight you will need daily exercise, and the ability to trust your body and natural instincts.

Fact:

Billions of dollars are spent annually, to conceal the facts about diet.

Knowing the difference between your optimal weight and ideal weight can help you lose weight also. Ideal weight is a common thought to many, which these people work to achieve a weight they fantasized in their mind. Optimal weight on the other hand, is what you are supposed to weight according to biochemical and genetic calculations.

When you reach your optimal weight you often feel good about you, and confident that you have achieved. Obsessed eaters often spend time trying to look like Arnold Swartznigger, or Faith Hill, that they lose track of reality. There is no way in the world you can look like someone you are not.

How you can stop obsessing is learning to accept who you are. Many women have been torn down by media, magazines, unruly men behaviors, and so forth. The damage leads them to fantasy about who they want to look like. These women often sit around daydreaming about who they want to look like and what they could do if they looked like that person.

While breakthroughs are showing the damage of media, faulty behaviors, thinking, slicks, and so forth, the fact is more damage has been done that what anyone can truly repair. Still, you can start now and live longer, happier, and healthier.

If you are obsessed with being thin, you are wasting your time, since if you accept your body now you have a head start to a better living. Life is too short to not enjoy you. When you learn to enjoy you, pamper self, and take time out for you, you can also grow to a healthier future. So what if you do not look like Cindy Crawford, who cares. Cindy will fade with the media, while you can live longer, healthier, and happier, by learning to accept and put obsession behind you...

Families are falling apart nowadays, thus we need a way to help them come together again.

CHAPTER 13- FAMILY GUIDE

Communication breakdowns cause emotional stress, which leads to major problems.

Families are falling apart nowadays. Relationships are blundering, and millions of people each day stress to find a way to find happiness. They often resort to cheating, lying, or acting out emotional in various ways. Instead of trying to find a solution, they often make excuses, thus millions of people are in denial as a result. Now we can sit down and talk about vitamins, nutrition, or magic pills that could persuade you to live longer, happier, and healthier. The fact is there is no magic pill that will help you; rather it takes you to make it happen. You need to consider your habits, behaviors, and lifestyle as a whole now.

Behaviors can spend our time, as well as cause us to fall apart. Often behaviors come from overwhelming stress, depression, and so forth. The stress and depression comes from negative thinking. Millions of people in the world spend time rehearsing what they will say and do, spar their thoughts, placate, or else fantasize about the way they prefer life to be. Most people derail, read minds, judge, and so forth, rather than letting go and letting God take care of business.

All the chaos leads to fighting, arguments, and breakdown in families. The problem is a breakdown in communication, responses of the emotions that take control, the way people think, and the way they act in between.

Dialect also plays a part in the many problems we face today. Dialect is our language, parlance, tongue, and the way we talk. When we phrase things, or say something we express our feelings but many people read minds. Dialect includes slang, jargons, argots, speech, and language. When you learn to understand dialect you will find it easier to communicate.

Communication breakdowns cause emotional stress, which leads to major health problems. The breakdowns in communication is breaking down friendships, families, and even causing major world issues for all of us. At the moment the United States Government is working with India to build communication, yet they are only working to build technological communication. We need effective communication, which includes listening, hearing, observing, and feeling. I feel what you are saying is common amongst black people. This is an outstanding quality these people present. Take note and follow pursuit, since when you feel what is said, you find deeper meaning and understanding.

When couples spend years together, they often fall apart due to various reasons. Some of the reason is they do not spend quality time, and they fail to communication. They will often spend time in fantasies wishing for something better, when better is often sitting in front of them.

Many people today cut off those speaking. This breaks down communication, which leads to problems. Messages are In between communications and if you listen without judging, or showing prejudice you will hear what those messages are sending. Often when the emotions take control and communication is misled, people take the easy way out by drinking excessively, using drugs, arguing, and fighting over things that mean nothing at all.

If you want to live healthier and longer you will need to change your habits. You will also need to deepen activities and learn how to express yourself properly.

Life is too short to spend time BSING around. Spend time learning to communicate, understanding dialect, and you will soon feel stress reduce, which in turn will bring you happiness. In summary, to live happier you will need proper thinking, exercise, and the eye to see what is in front of you when it hits.

Chapter 14- Understanding the Healthier Lifestyle

Learning effective communication techniques will guarantee you a life that is healthier and happier.

Down through the century's lies has spread throughout the lands, accordingly downgrading our system. We have advantages today, since men in white coats are spending time to find ways to help you (them) live longer, healthier, and happier, yet they are still walking around with blind folds on. Sure, they are getting a deeper understanding, yet they fail to hear the truths. Still, we must learn that exercise is a part of the problem as well; rather lack of exercise is causing major problems. Exercise will jack up the musculoskeletal system.

Did you not know that instincts were given to you at birth? Did you not know that those instincts could guide you better than any man in the world? Did you know that down through the centuries, man has distorted natural instincts?

Down through the years people has told you that if you adhere to this diet plan you can lose weight, which will make you feel good and happier. The fact is no diet plan in the world will work for most people, since they live to be someone they are not.

Instincts can guide you to better health, yet most people will ignore natural instincts. For instance, something told me not to go to the bar last night. Yet, the person may go anyway and wonder why he is in jail the next day.

If you allow nature to take its course, you will see the right path to follow. Still, you need to build wisdom to take you far and wide.

Wisdom is perceptions and intelligence. When you use wisdom to make decisions you use good judgment, while forming penetrating thoughts that helps you to see clearly. Wisdom promotes good sense. You achieve wisdom through knowledge, understanding, insight, and so forth.

One of the reasons people are stressing over living longer, healthier, and happier is because many feel the world is ready to end. They fear death and they believe that if they change their ways now, they can live longer. The fact is you can, yet when Judgment Day comes, it may be too late. Still, you want to use good sense from here on out to live healthier.

Good sense includes exercise. The body composes metabolism, bones, muscles, joints, cells, tissues, tendons, ligaments, nerves, and more. One of the best things I learnt in life is if you take care of your muscles and joints, you will live a healthier life.

The one thing you want to take care of is your cardiovascular system, respiratory system, nervous system, gastrointestinal system, musculoskeletal system, integumentary system, hematologic and lymphatic system, endocrine system, and sensory and motor systems.

Most of the diseases that occur today come from lack of exercise. The musculoskeletal systems are essential. The skeleton includes about 206 bones. The bones are long, flat, short, and irregular. The musculoskeletal system includes calcium, phosphorus, magnesium, and the bone marrow produces RBCS (Red blood cells).

The muscles work to give us support, enables us to move, and protects our eternal organs. The muscles work to allow the body to move freely through relaxation and contractions while working the posture through tightening and shortening the muscles.

Exercise is the only solution that will protect this valuable system, thus if you want to live healthier, longer, and happier put those muscles to work. As you can see using your instincts, combined with exercise and learning effective communication you can live longer, healthier, and happier. Still, you need spiritual food, which only comes from the bible and mediation. You want to be careful because many religions have misled people for centuries. Understanding musculoskeletal systems and exercise and how they work together can help you live healthier.

CHAPTER 15- THE MUSCULOSKELETAL SYSTEM AND EXERCISE

When you maintain proper weight on the muscles and reduce stress on the joints, you will be happier ans healthier in the long run.

Many people fail to see how exercise can benefit the musculoskeletal system, which can help them live healthier, longer, and happier. The musculoskeletal system is the body's anatomy ad physiological aspects of the body. The skeleton is part of this system, which comprises of 206 long, flat, short, and irregular bones. The skeleton stores calcium, phosphorus, magnesium, and the bone marrow is what produce the red blood cells.

The muscles work to prove support, as well as locomotion, and all while protecting the internal organs.

The skeletal muscles provide us posture and movement, which tightens and shortens as the muscles attach to the bones through tendons. The muscles start to contract as stimulus of the muscles fiber reaches the motor neurons. The production leads to energy, which produces muscle contraction, which stems from the hydrolysis which comes from ATP (Adenosine Triphosphate) and spreads to the ADP (Adenosine Diphosphate) and then moves to the phosphate.

The muscles also retain contractions, which maintain the tone of muscle. The muscles relax, which breakdowns of acetylcholine through cholinesterase occurs. The ligaments attach to the muscles, which are tough bands of collagen fibers, which attaches to the bones. The system encircles the joints that add stability and strength.

Elaine Owens

The tendons attach, which tendons are non-elastic cords of collagen. The tendons attach to the muscles and the bones. The joints attach to the tendons, which the articulate surfaces joints two bones. The joints provide stability, and allow us to move. Joints offer a degree of movement, which is known as ROM (Range of Motion)

The joints also attach to synovium, which are the membranes where the joints line the inner surface of the muscles. Synovium secretes synovial fluids, which include antibodies. (Pain Fighters) Synovium reduces the friction within the joints, which are in conjunction of the cartilages.

The cartilages serve as smooth surfaces that articulate the bones and absorb joint shock, which atrophies alongside limited ROM, will affect the weight bearing joints that often lead to problems.

Bursa is a fluid-filled sac, which serves to pad and reduce friction. Bursa facilitates motion of the body's structure, which rubs against the other.

What we discussed is the musculoskeletal system, alongside reasons that the systems are damaged. For the most part exercise plays a large part, i.e. lack of movement of the muscles. When the body does not get exercise, pain, stiffness, numbness, fatigue, fevers, swelling, and immobility occur. This leads to serious complications, especially if something isn't done soon. Often when a person does not exercise the skin breaks down, ROM is limited, edema sets in, inflammatory occurs, muscle spasms happen, and the list goes on.

To prevent problems you need to learn to relax and flex the muscles to promote healthier joints. What happens is when you exercise you start to feel better, since stress is released; disease is limited, and so forth. If you fail to do exercise you will suffer serious health problems later, and in time you will die younger than you were expected. One thing you want to learn about exercise is that you want to avoid placing high volumes of stress on the joints. The muscles are what you want to build or strengthen.

When you maintain proper weight on the muscles and reduce stress on the joints, you can live happier, healthier, and longer. Taking care of the musculoskeletal system will lead you to a happier road in life. Now think positive energy!

CHAPTER 16- POSITIVE ENERGY

When you have a positive mindset, you are on the path to achieving your goals.

Positive energy sends out messages that will make others listen. On top of this, positive energy is the choice that will make you live longer, healthier, and happier. Positive comes from brains that think optimistic. The brain is constructive and helpful in assisting a productive response. When a person thinks positive they feel encouraged, and will use affirmatives to lead their path.

Positive energy comes from activists who live it up by adhering to an upbeat attitude. They avoid negative thinking at all cost.

Positive energy will make you feel certain, while clearing up issues that come your way. You are convinced, which assures you that what you say and do, and how you look is ok with you. Positive energy is definite. Nothing can break those with positive energy, since they are explicit in all areas of their life. The positive thinkers are clear-cut and to the point. These people use conclusive thinking to resolve problems, and clear up unquestionable areas. The positive energy leads them to make sound decisions.

Where Do I Get Positive Energy?

You dig deep inside you and stop fighting yourself. When you instincts and emotions tell you something, listen instead of jumping to conclusions. You get positive energy when you hang around positive influences, and stop judging, criticizing, or acting out of bias thoughts. You fight for what you believe, since you will go to lengths to prove what you believe has facts to verify what you say. You have convictions that no man, woman, child, or anyone can stand against.

Understanding positive thinking can help you find energy that leads to positive results. When you think the world has you down, look around, and you will see the world is only getting those down who allow it to happen. When you have negative thoughts it promotes quicker death. How? Well, let's consider.

Negative energy is a major killer. When a person thinks negative he shows no enthusiastic in life. Often the person will act out destructively. The person's thoughts are often unhelpful, and lead to procrastination, laziness, downbeat, depression, harm, damage, and finally destruction. Overall, denial sums up those who think negative. These people refuse to see the truth although a wealth of evidence sits in front of them.

Positive energy on the other hand, will help you to live longer, healthier, and happier, as well as make you shine like a star on a hot summer night.

Fact:

Did you know that if the stars are out at night, the sun will shine the next day. We do not need weathermen to tell us what kind of day we are going to have. When you think positive you set your mind to accomplish. You know that you can do anything you choose to do, and often you will do what you want within reason. You can tell you now that you intend to live longer, healthier, and happier and bet tomorrow you will start action that will lead you to the goal. Just remember however that living healthier makes you live longer, in turn you find happiness.

Now set your mind:

I intend to exercise tomorrow:

Affirm: I want to live longer, healthier, and happier and I am going to achieve my goal.

Say: I accept me for who I am and I am not bothered with becoming someone else, since I am special and unique.

Verify: I am special and unique, because no one can be like me.

I deserve to live healthier, longer, and happier.

Keep moving to positive energy and exercise and I promise you, you will live longer, healthier and happier.

CONCLUSION

We've discussed diet, instinctive eaters, obsessed eaters, supplements, exercise, positive thinking, negative energy, and more. We hope that you take the information and verify the facts by practicing each day what you learned. In conclusion, we would like to thank you for reading all 3 Volumes and hope that you live healthier, longer, and happier. NOTE: Always keep your doctors' appointments, and never give up. When you think you had enough take some time out and live it up. Learn to relax and reduce stress. By exercising and thinking positively, you are on the road to a healthy life.

ABOUT THE AUTHOR

I knew there had to be more that I could be doing in my life to feel better about myself in general. I think the older we get, the more we want to live longer; but with a better quality of life of course. Living longer and not feeling well at the same time has a way of cheating longevity and happiness. The younger we are when we recognize this is the sooner we can start making decisions that in the long run will indeed make us live longer, be happier and healthier too.

The information mentioned in my books is just a way to motivate people, young or old, to make decisions that will positively impact their happiness, health and ultimately, longevity. I wish I would've known to consider these things a long time ago. But I felt it was important to write about them so that I can help my friends and others as well.